I0436274

Chubby Art Cartoon Colouring Book of Erotica

by
Alison Galvan

Copyright © 2016 Alison Galvan

All rights reserved.

ISBN-10: 1530741017
ISBN-13: 978-1530741014

DEDICATION

This one is for all you who have imagination, a twinkle in your eye and hearts full of laughter.
Enjoy!

WHAT IS EROTICA?

In its basic sense, erotica is literature or art dealing with sexual love. But delving more deeply, erotica is the philosophical contemplation on the aesthetics of sexual desire, sensuality and romantic love.
When we respect ourselves and our partners all sexual experience is positive, and positively erotic!

ACKNOWLEDGMENTS

As strange as this may sound, this being a book of erotica, but for this one I want to thank my pretty girl, my one and only beautiful daughter. She is the one who jumps around the kitchen with me screaming when things go well, and the one who gives me hugs and cheers me up when they don't. I am so proud and happy for her and all her success. She inspires me to keep going towards my goals as artist, author and entrepreneur.
Together we are an unbeatable winning team.
Love that Girl!

LICK MY HEART

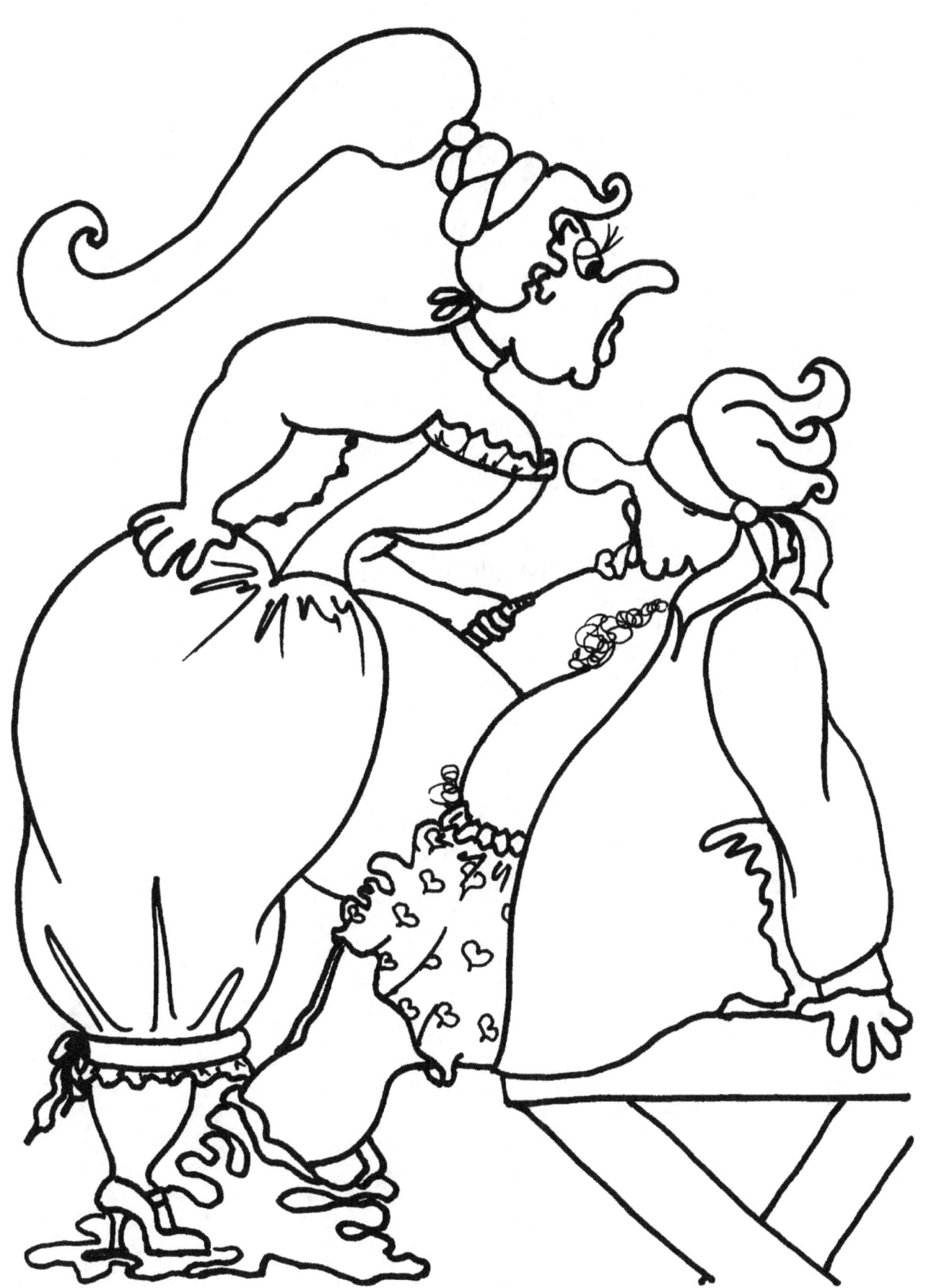

SWINGING 69

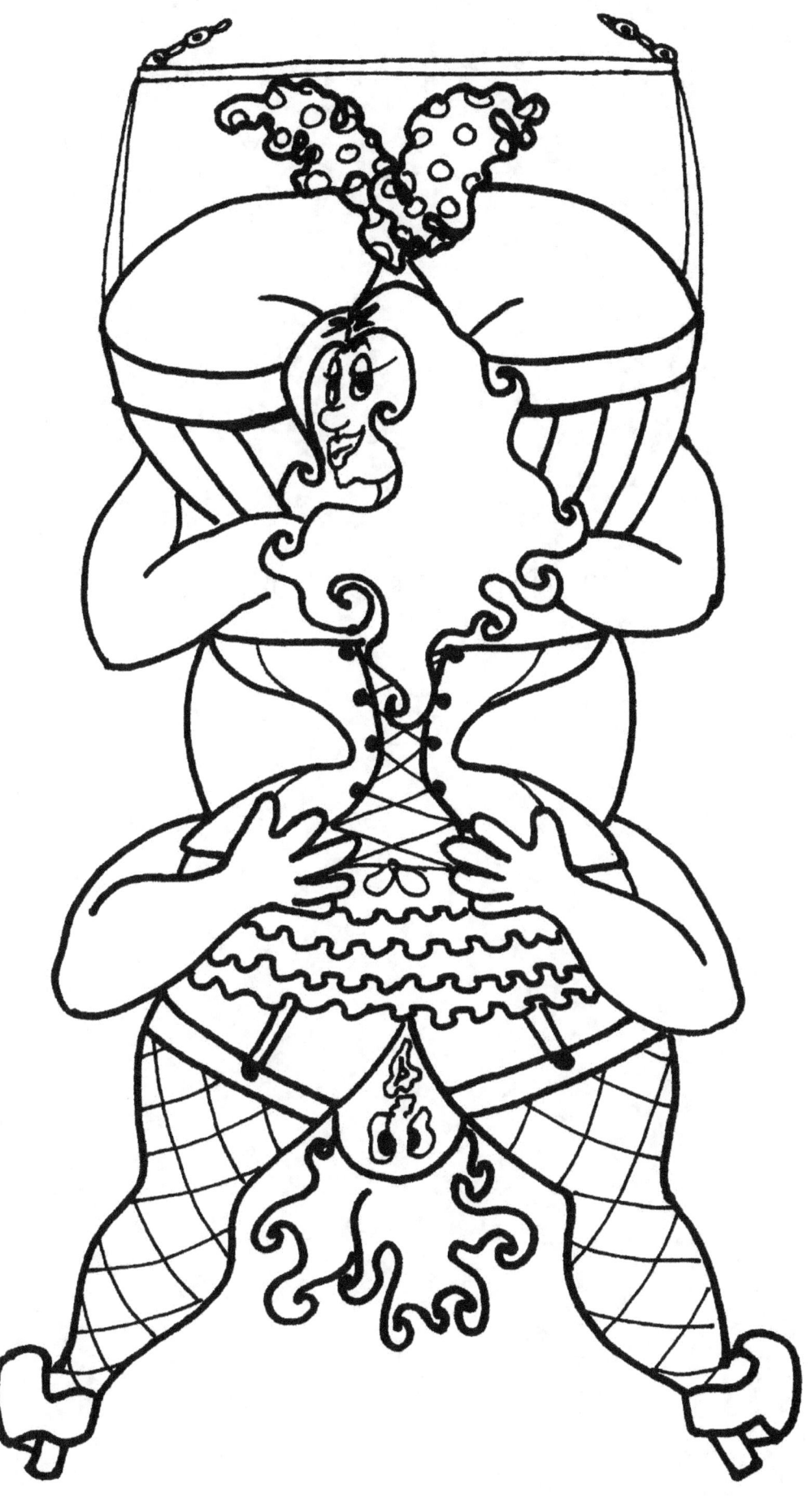

Alison Galvan

50 SHADES OF COLOURING

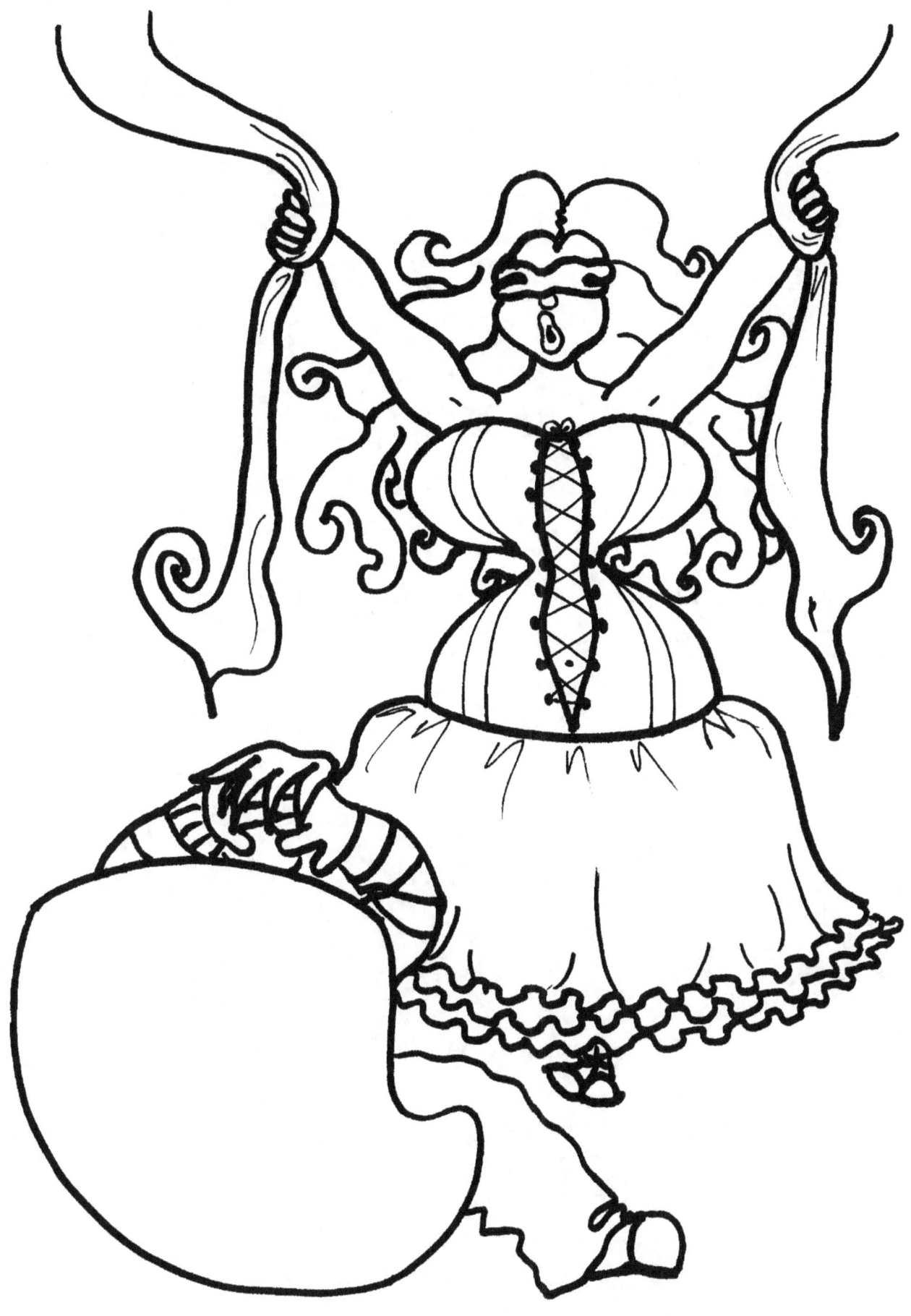

YOU ARE NEVER TOO OLD.... FOR A PROPELLER BRA!

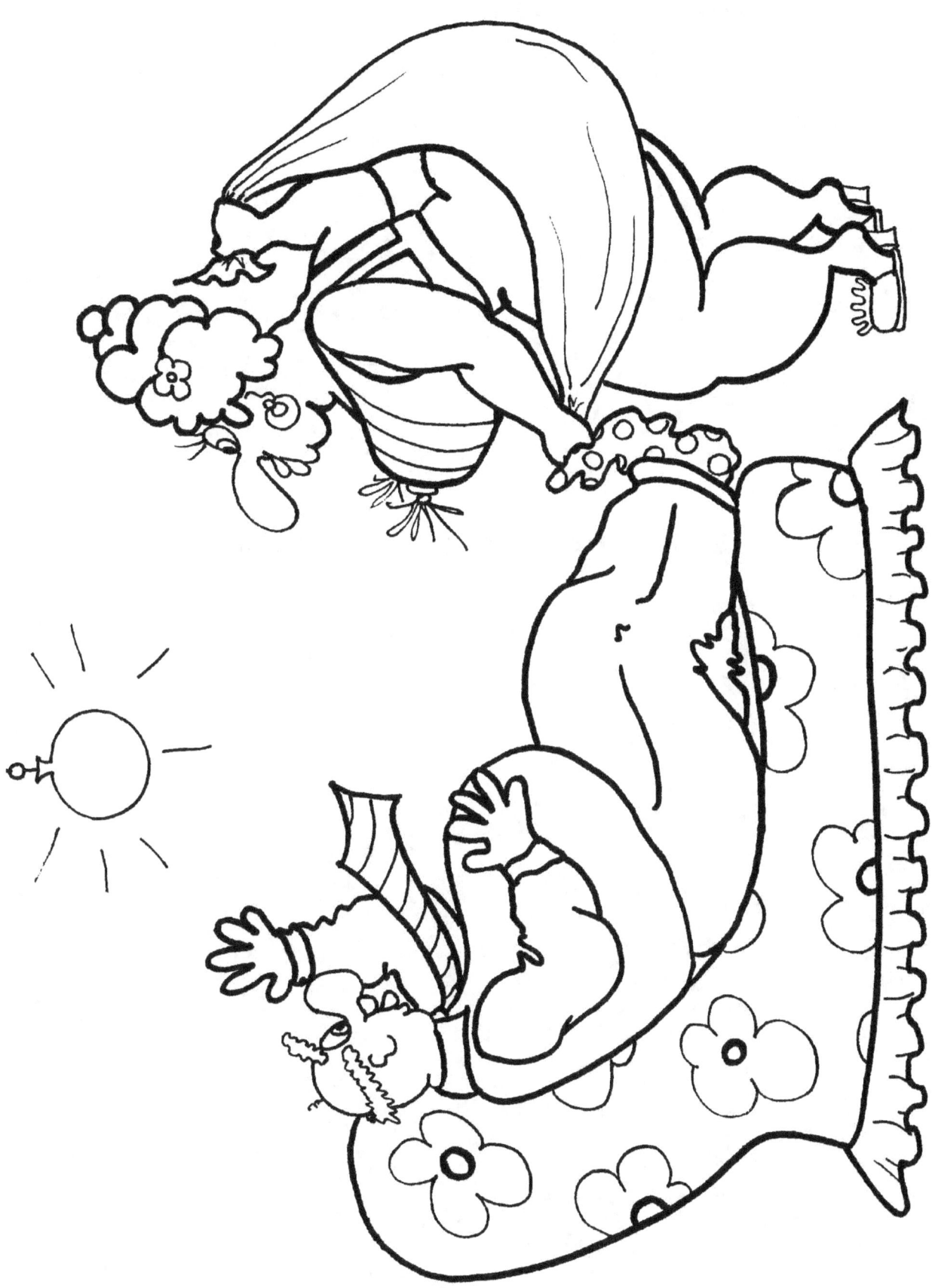

STRAWBERRIES AND CHAMPAGNE

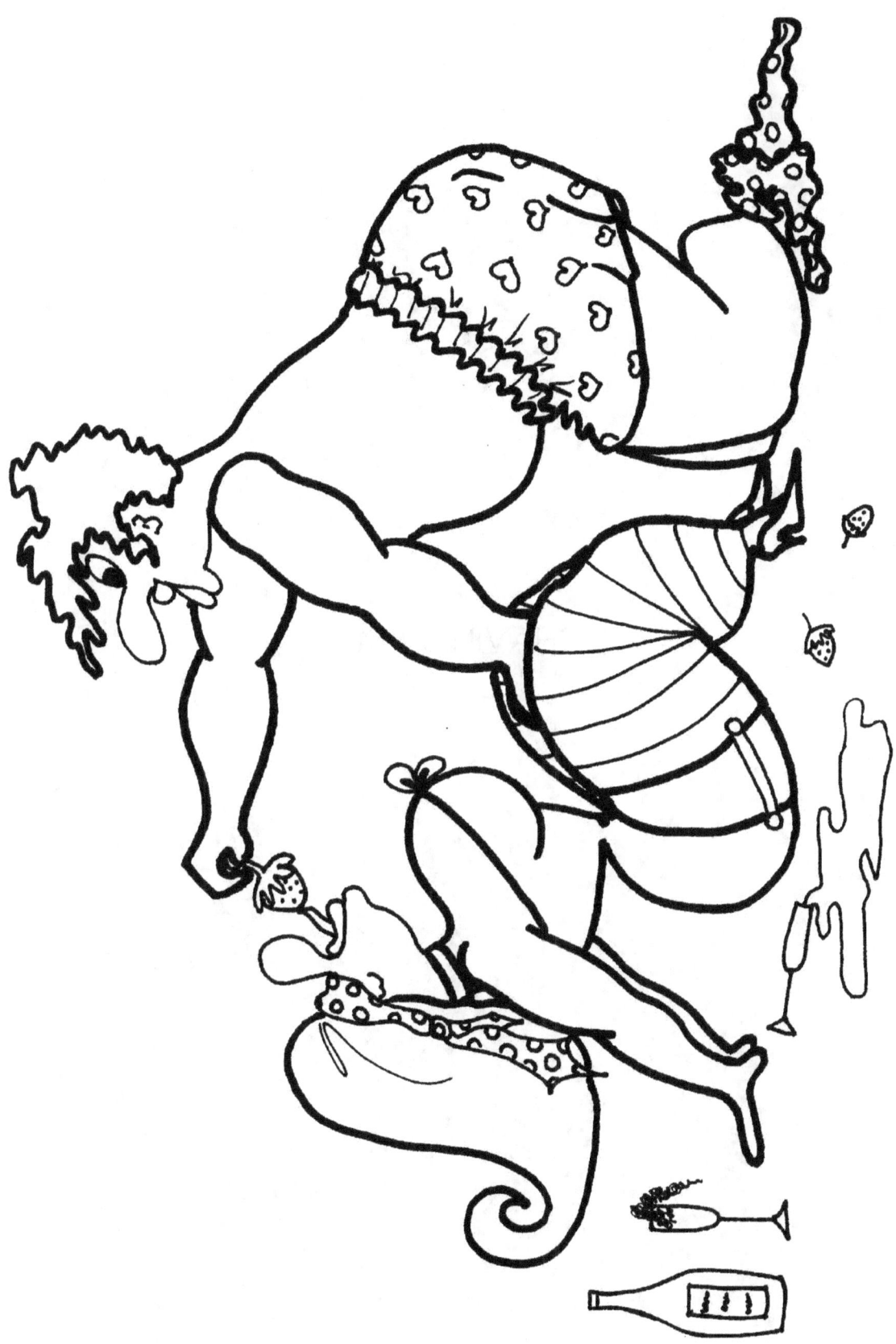

SHAVING TIME

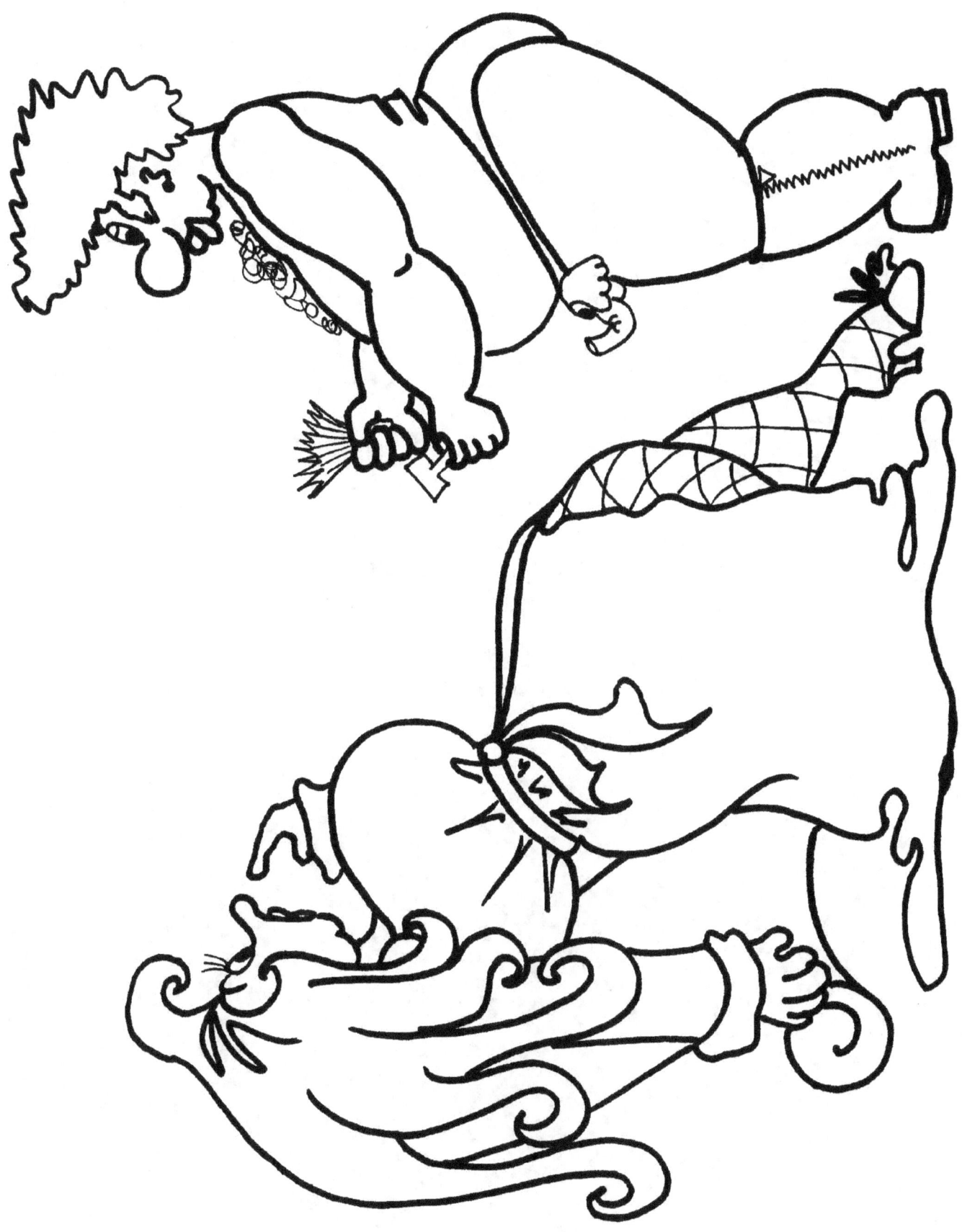

WEAVE MY BASKET

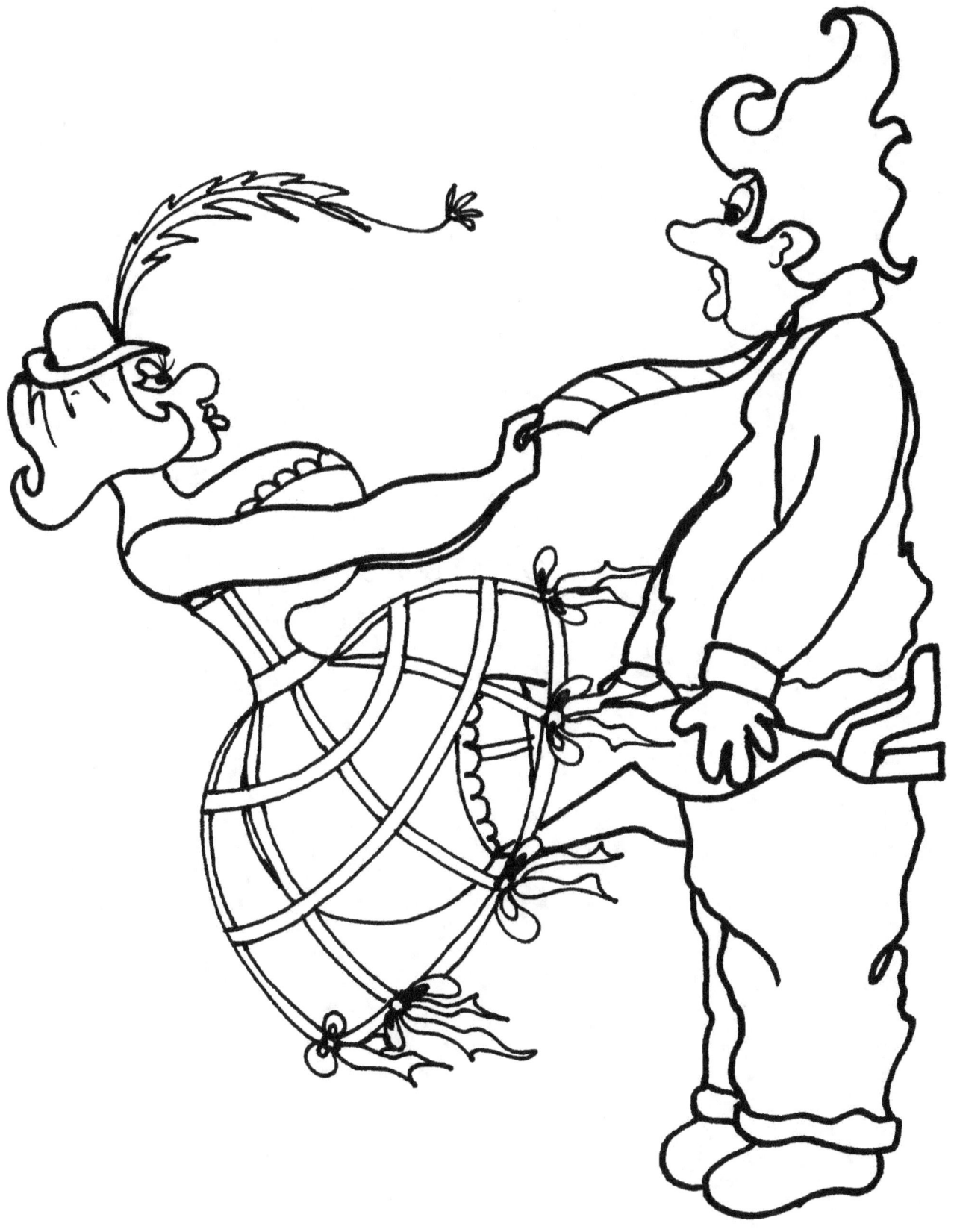

Alison Galvan

GIDDY-UP BOYS

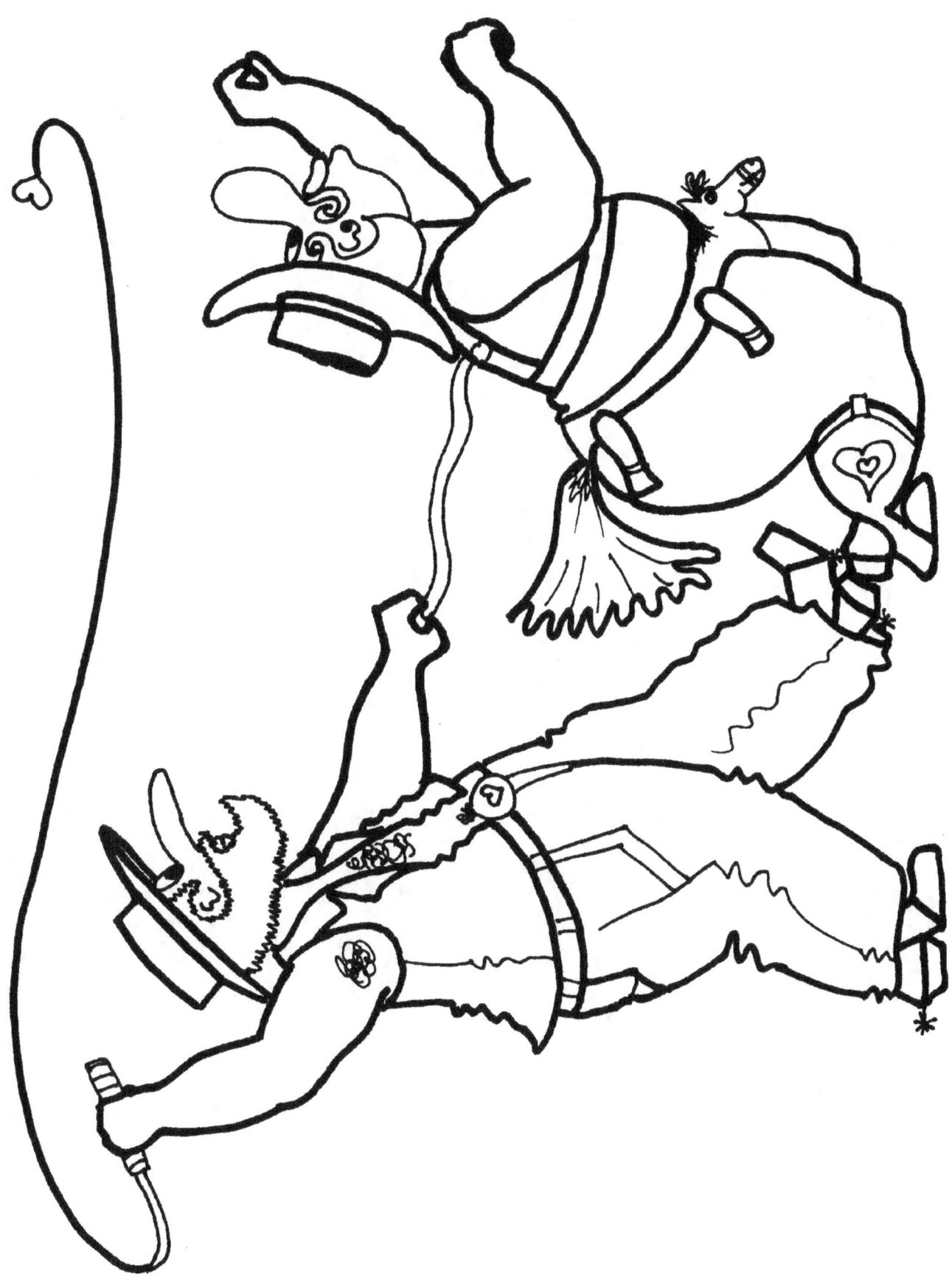

ALL TOGETHER NOW!

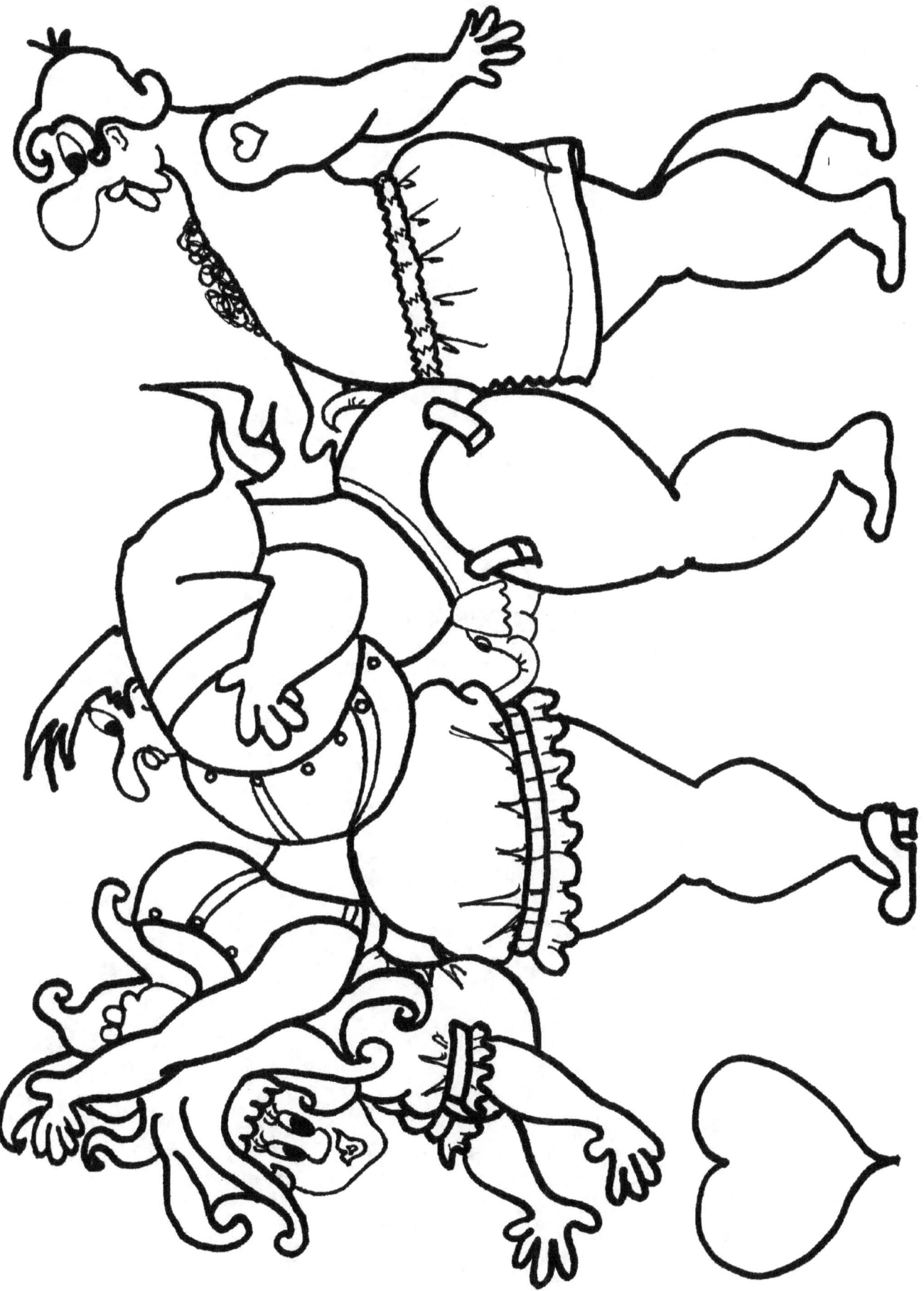

A TO DO IN THE LOO!

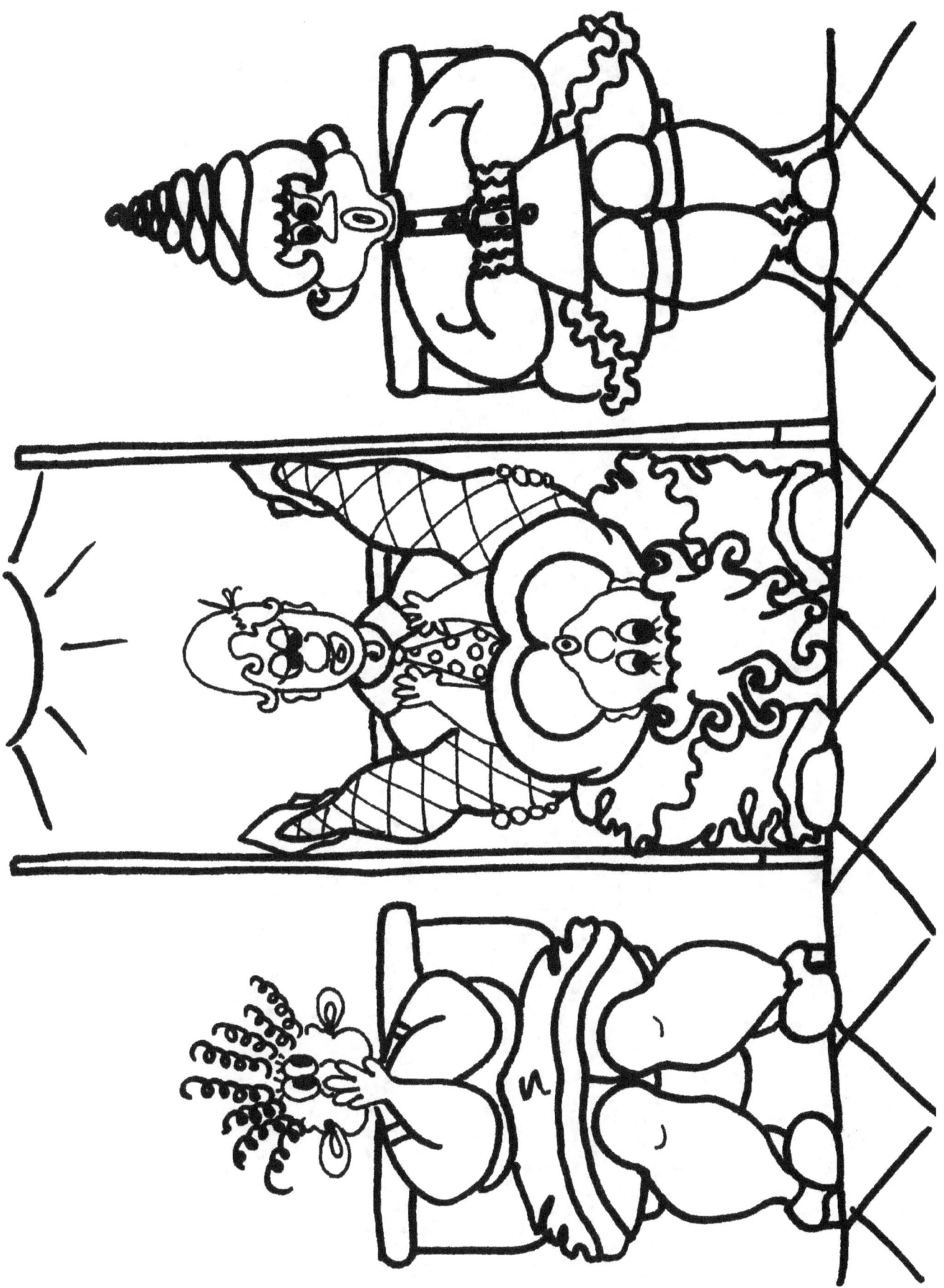

NOW THAT'S LOVE!

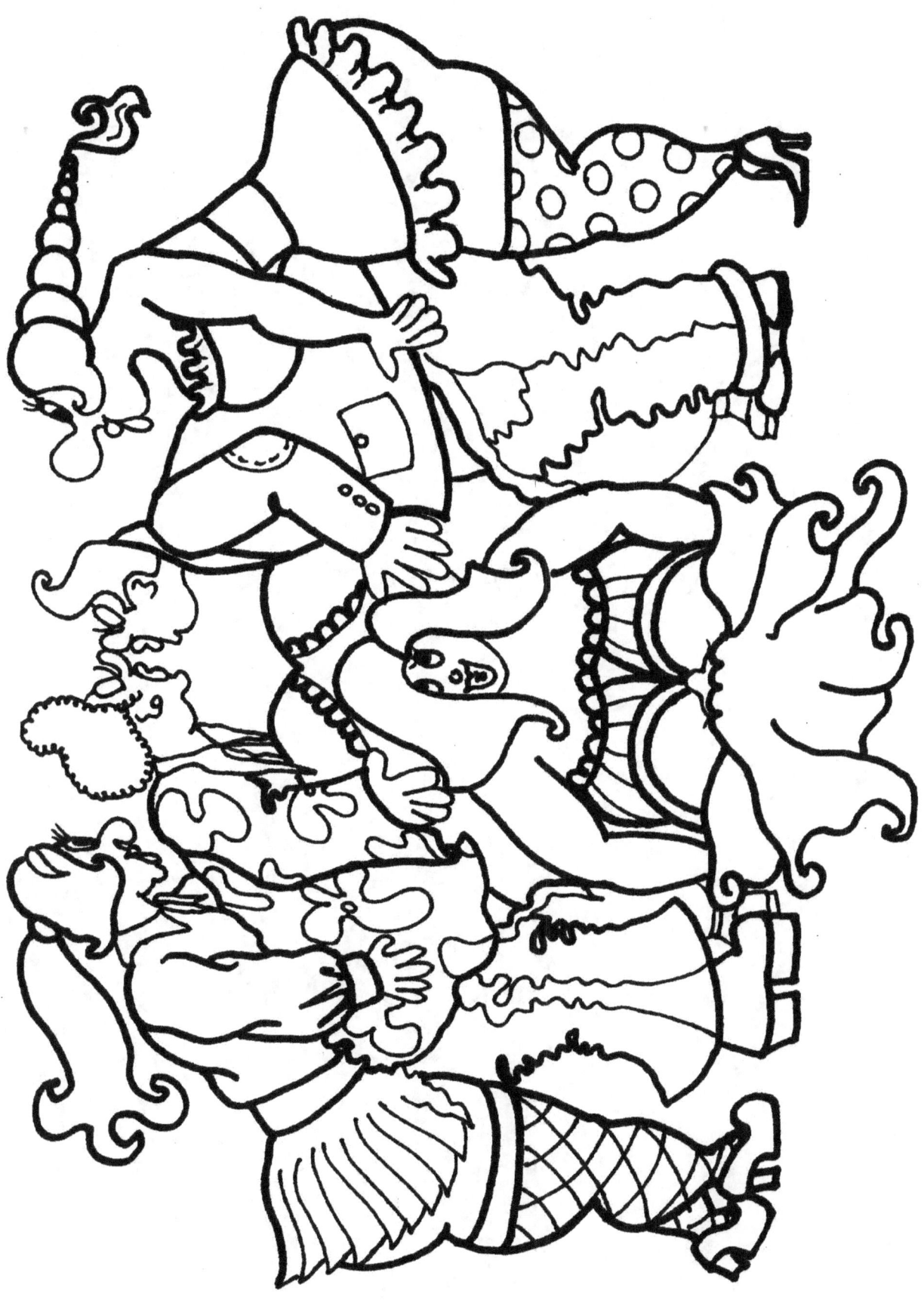

FANTASY FORCE

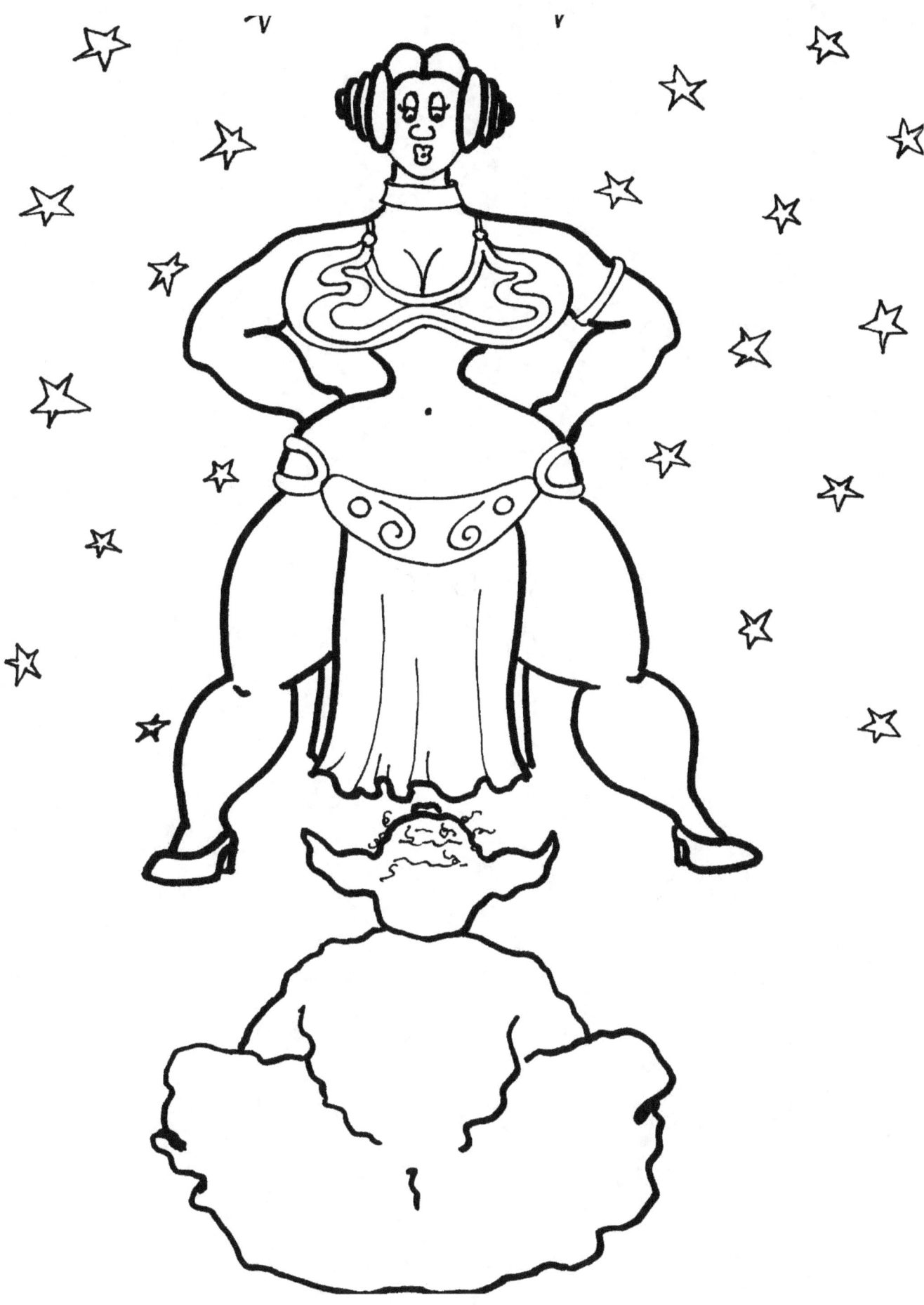

ADORATION

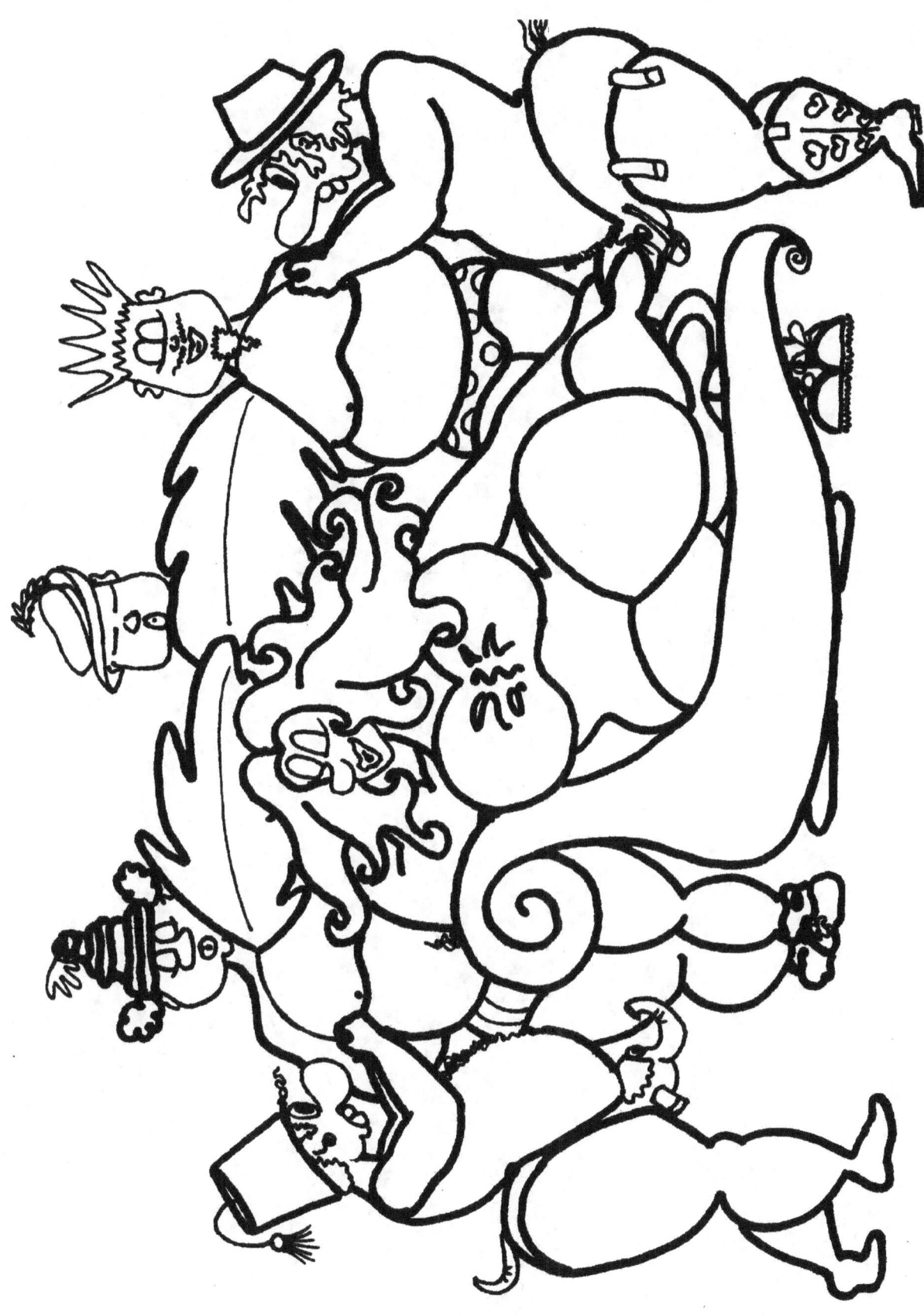

BLOWING UP THE BATHROOM

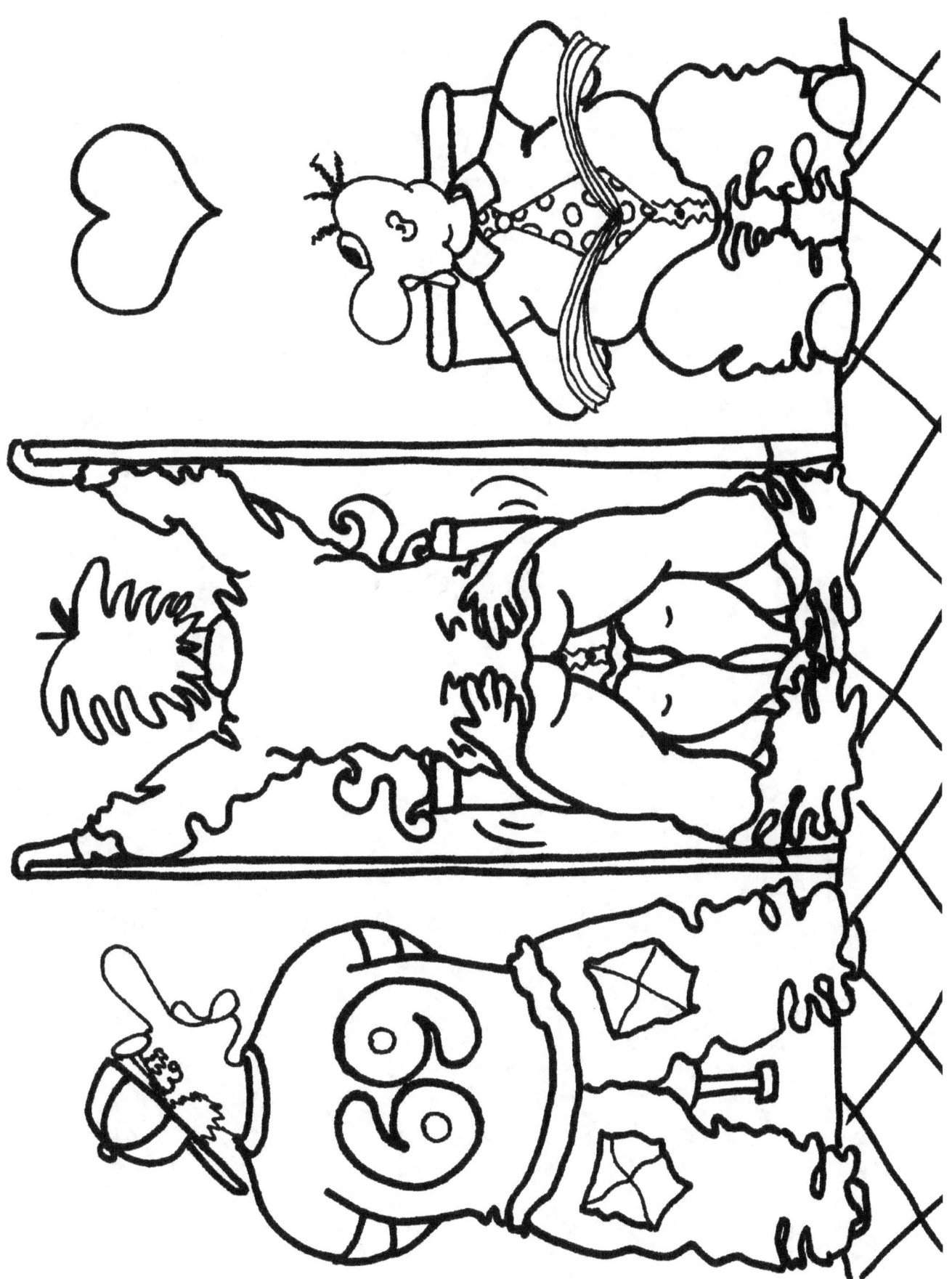

STRIP POKER

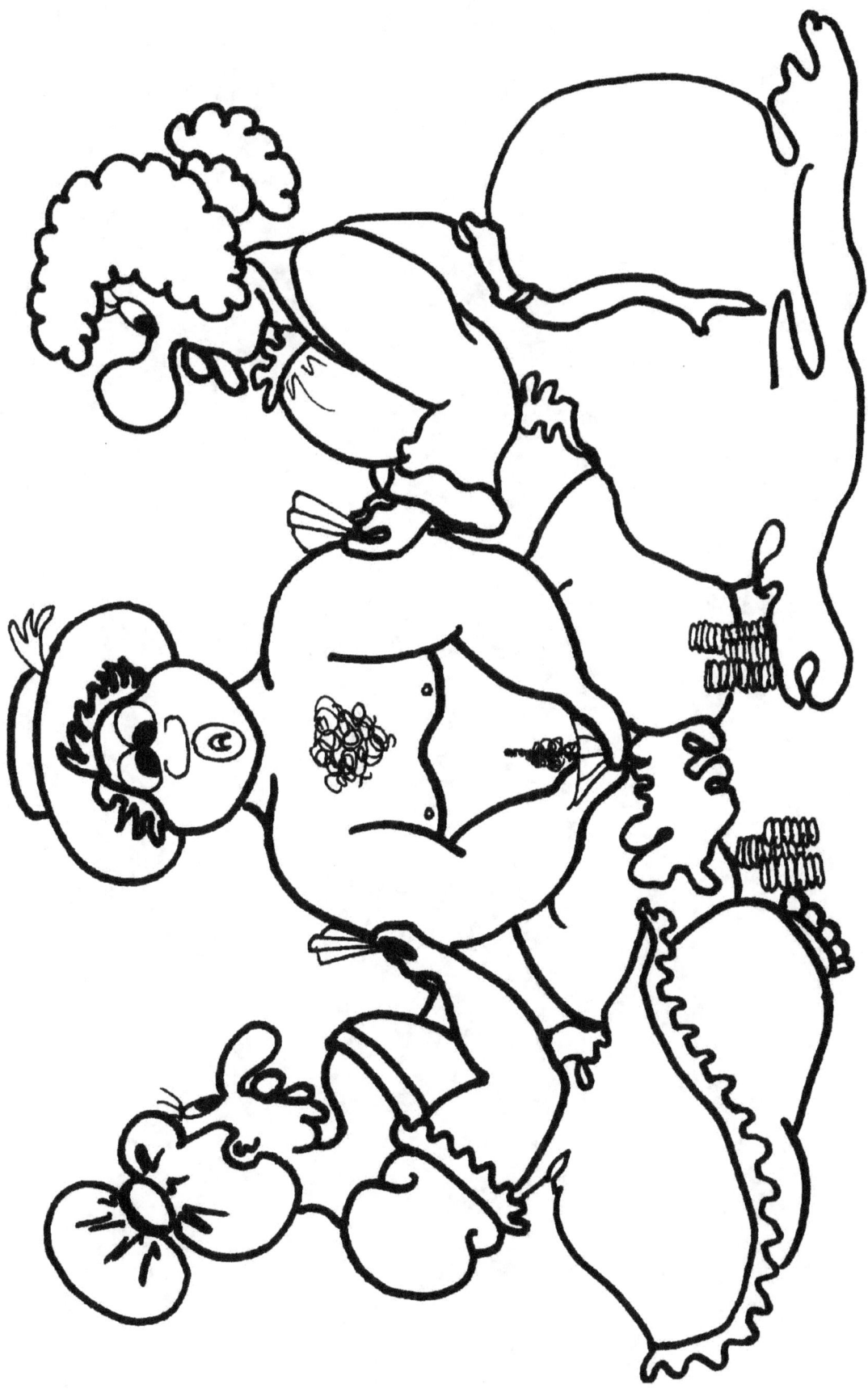

TICKLE MY TUSHY

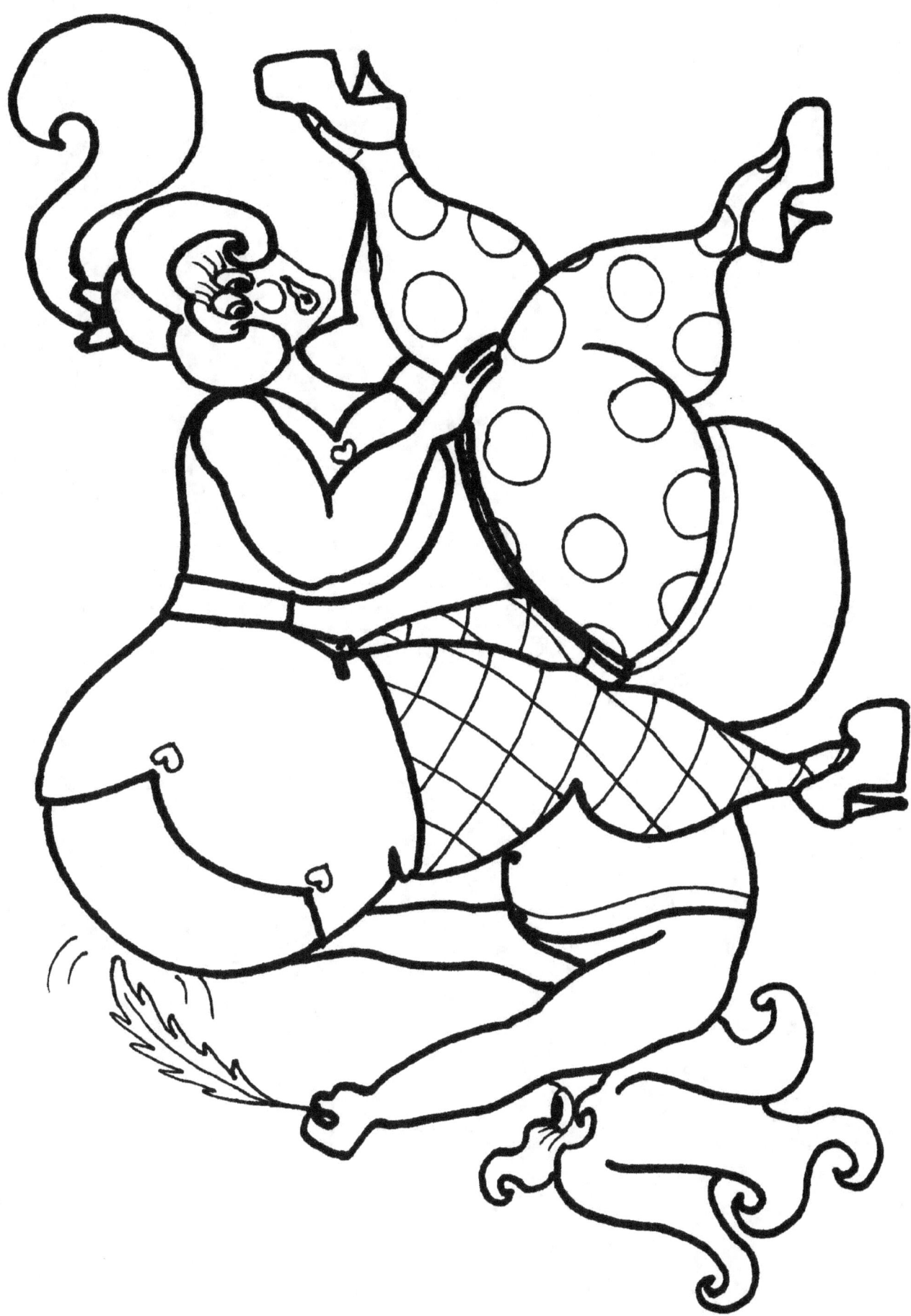

KISS MY CHUBBY

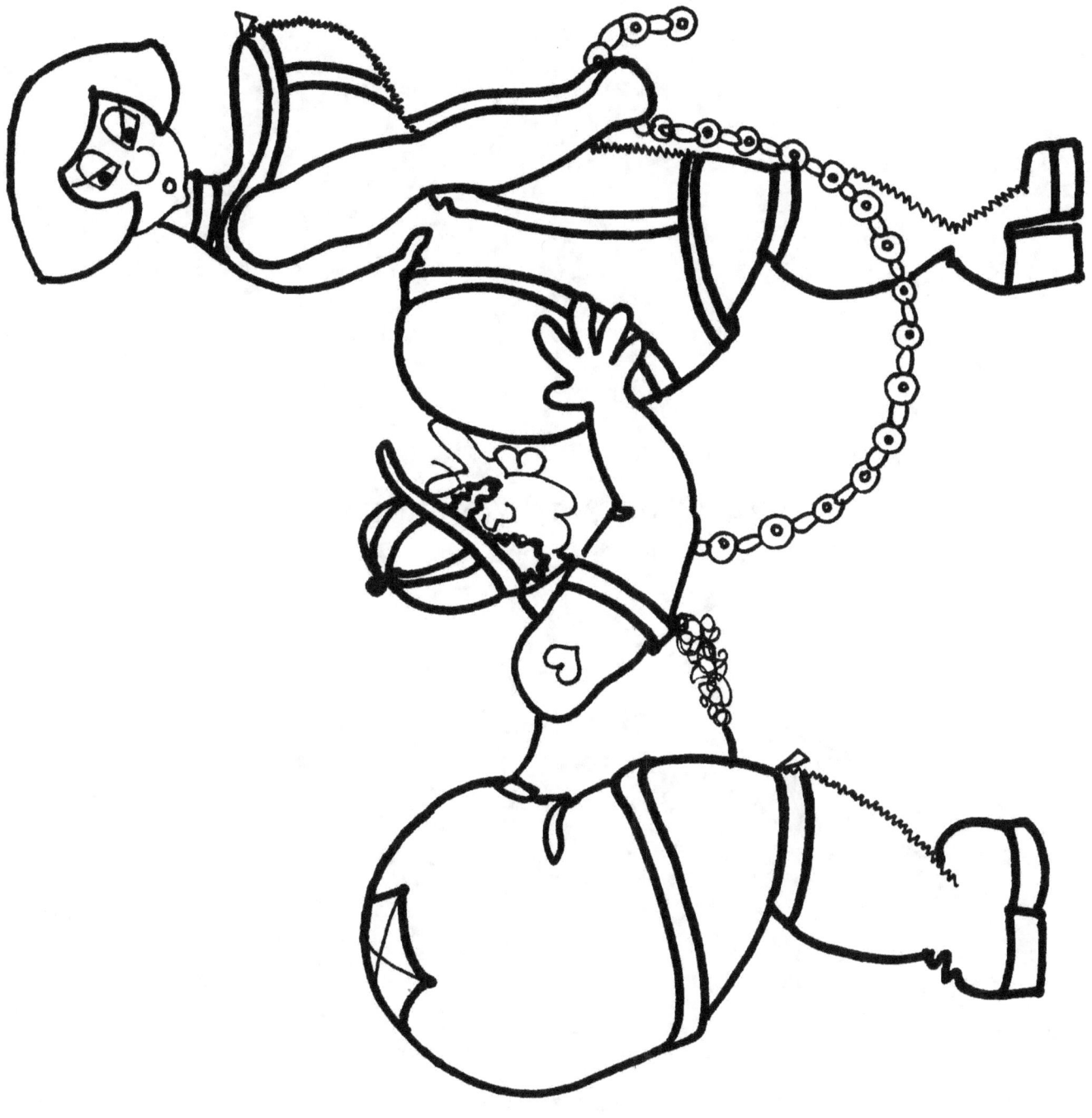

SPANK ME WITH YOUR HEART

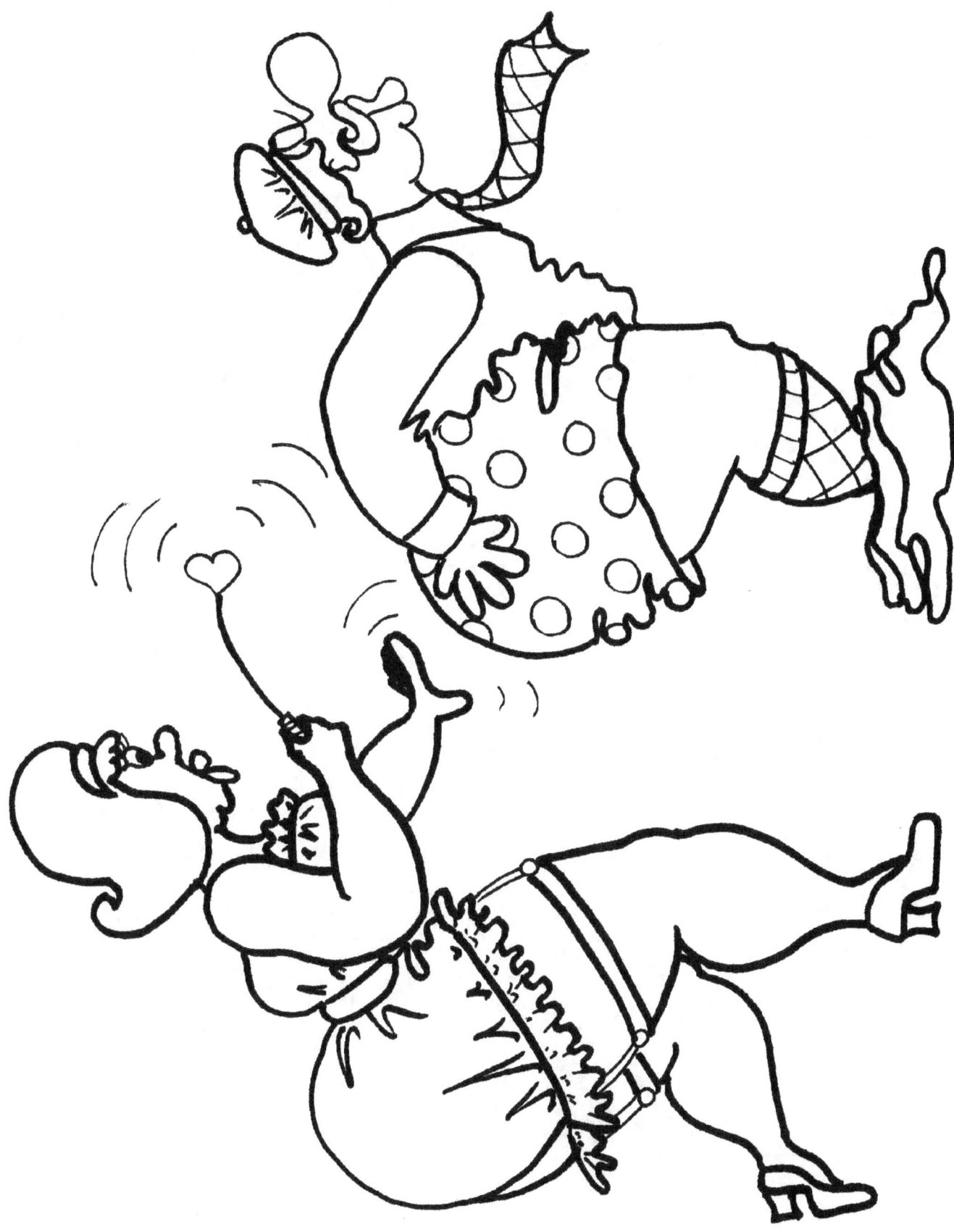

PAINTED TOENAILS

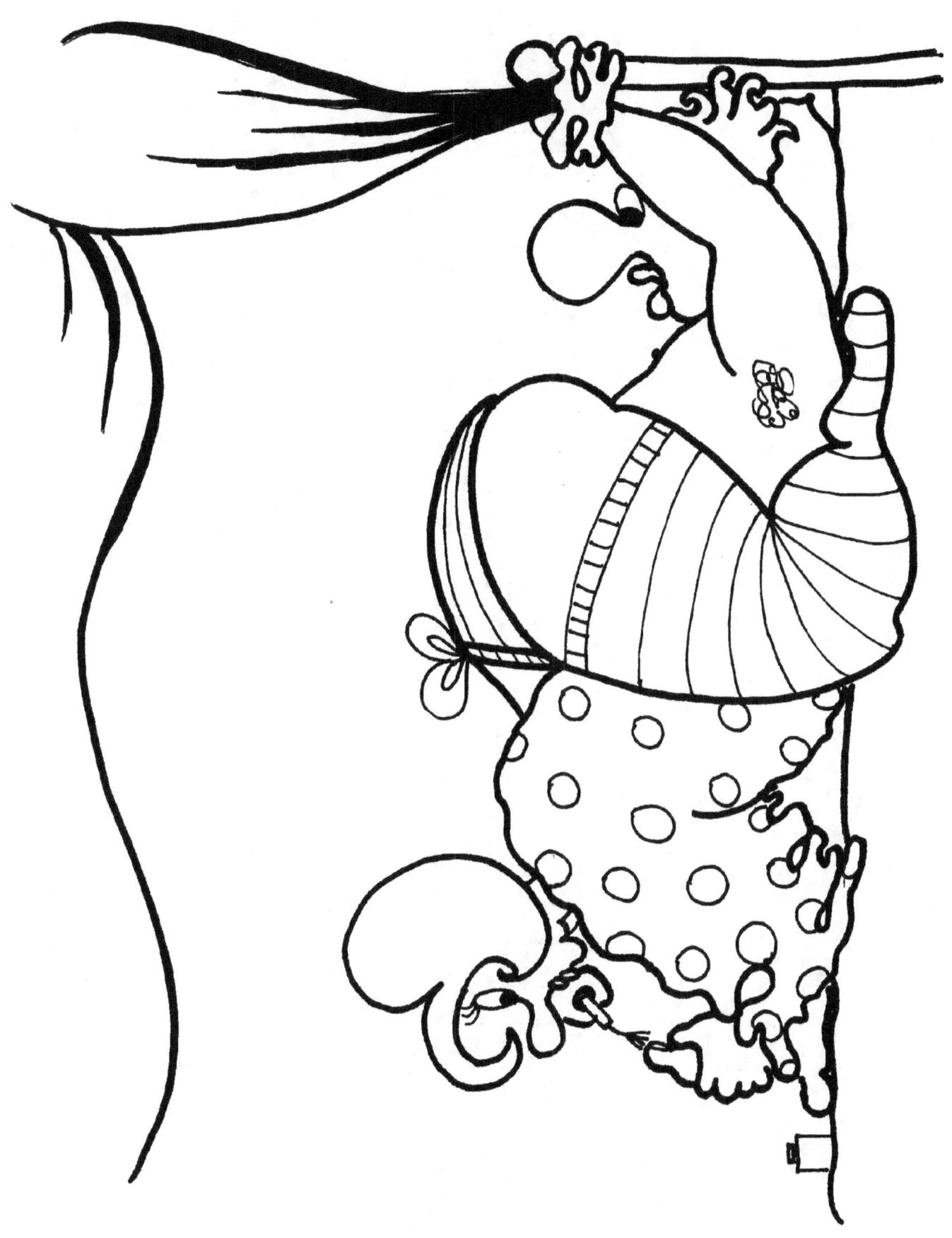

SPANK ME BABY!

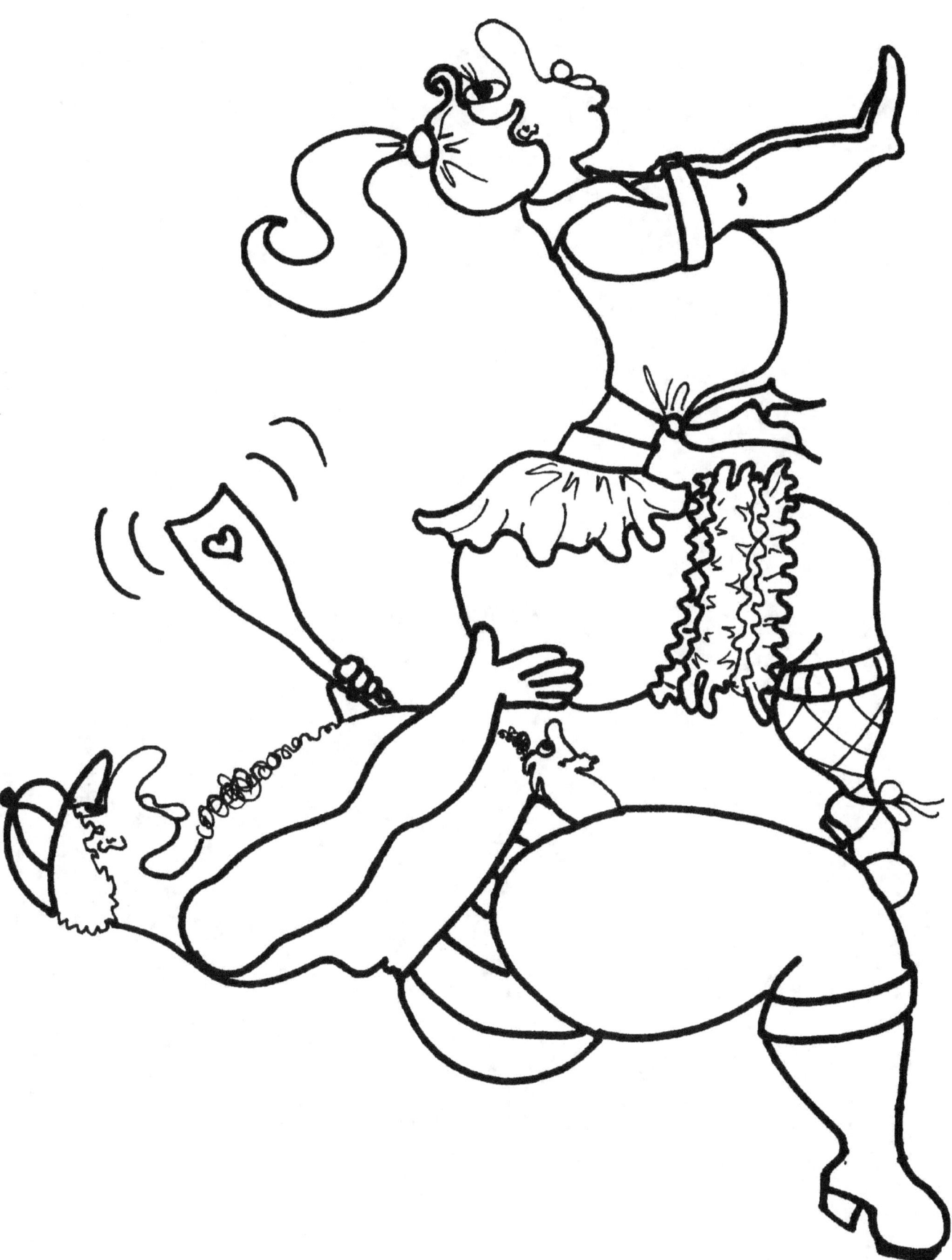

Alison Galvan

FEATHER TIME

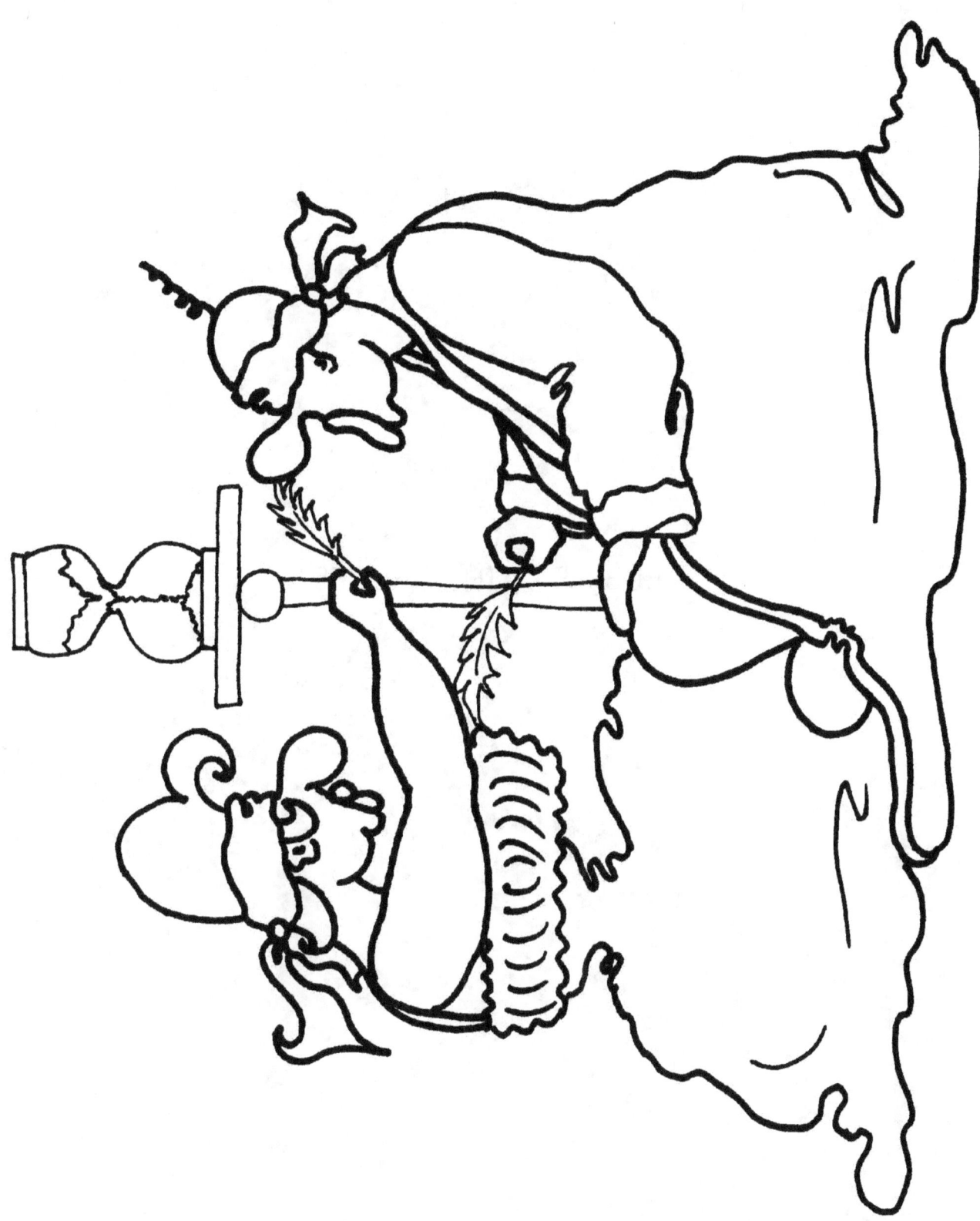

BUBBLE BATH BEAUTIES

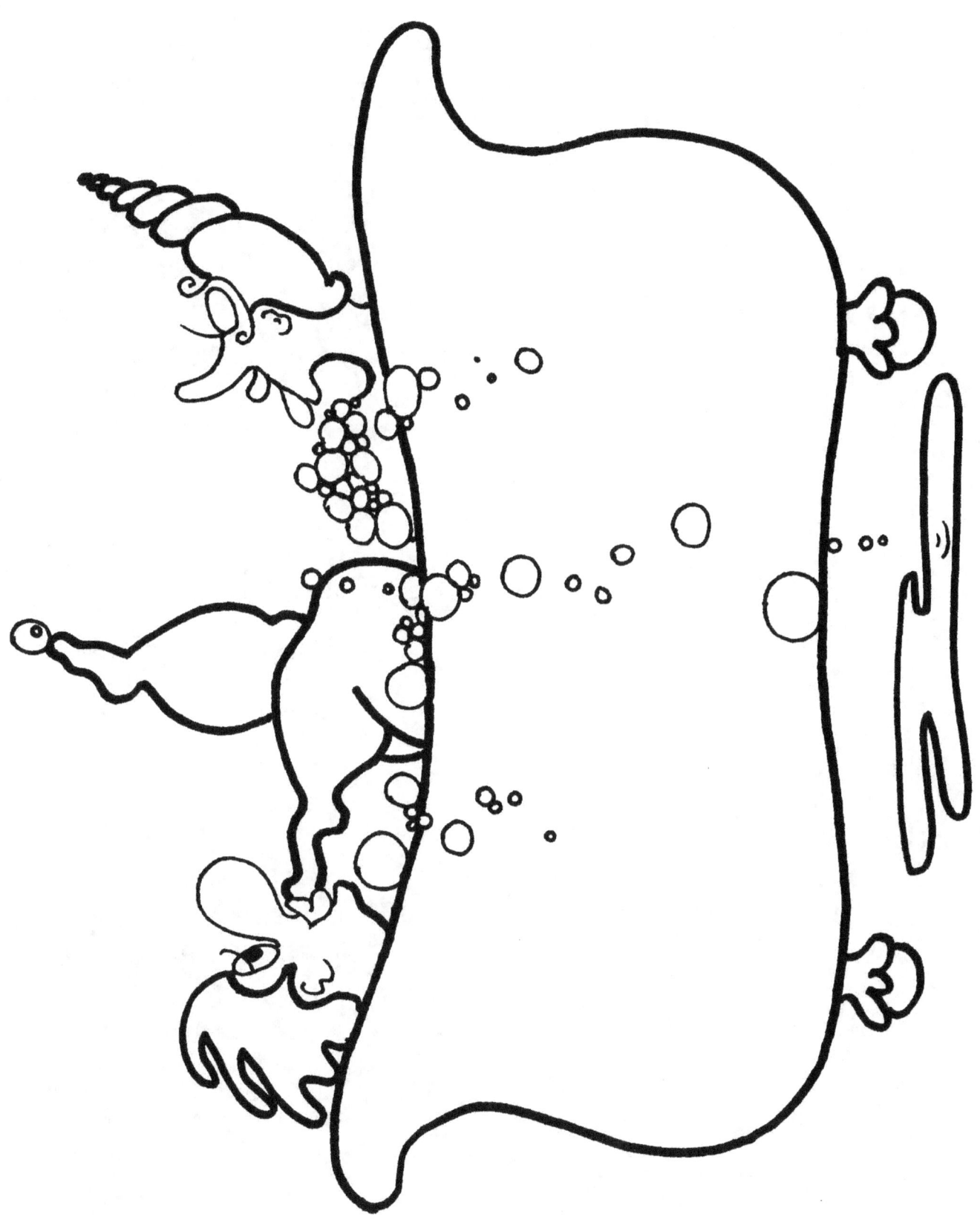

SWINGING IN REVERSE

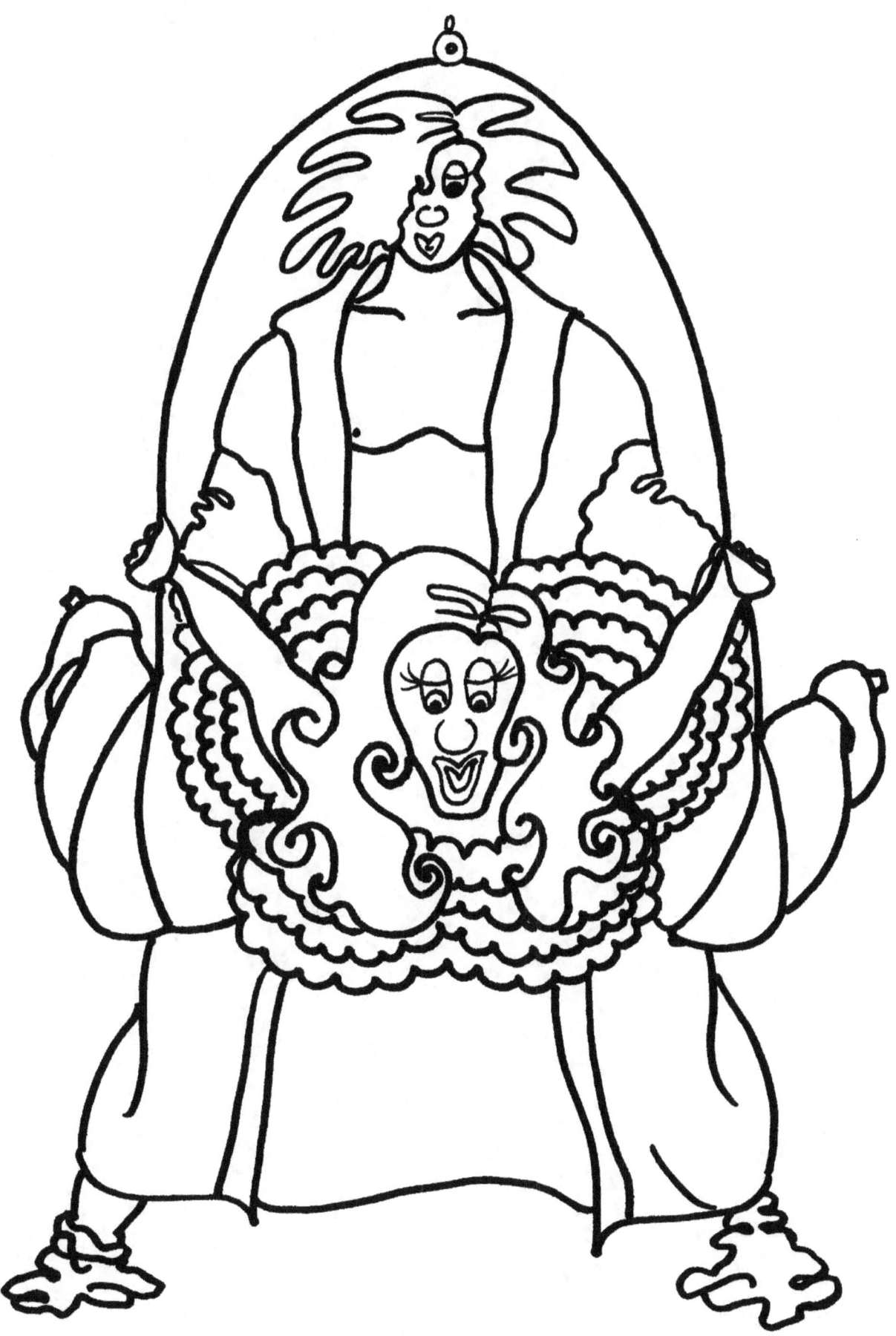

GLADIATOR STRIPPER BOY

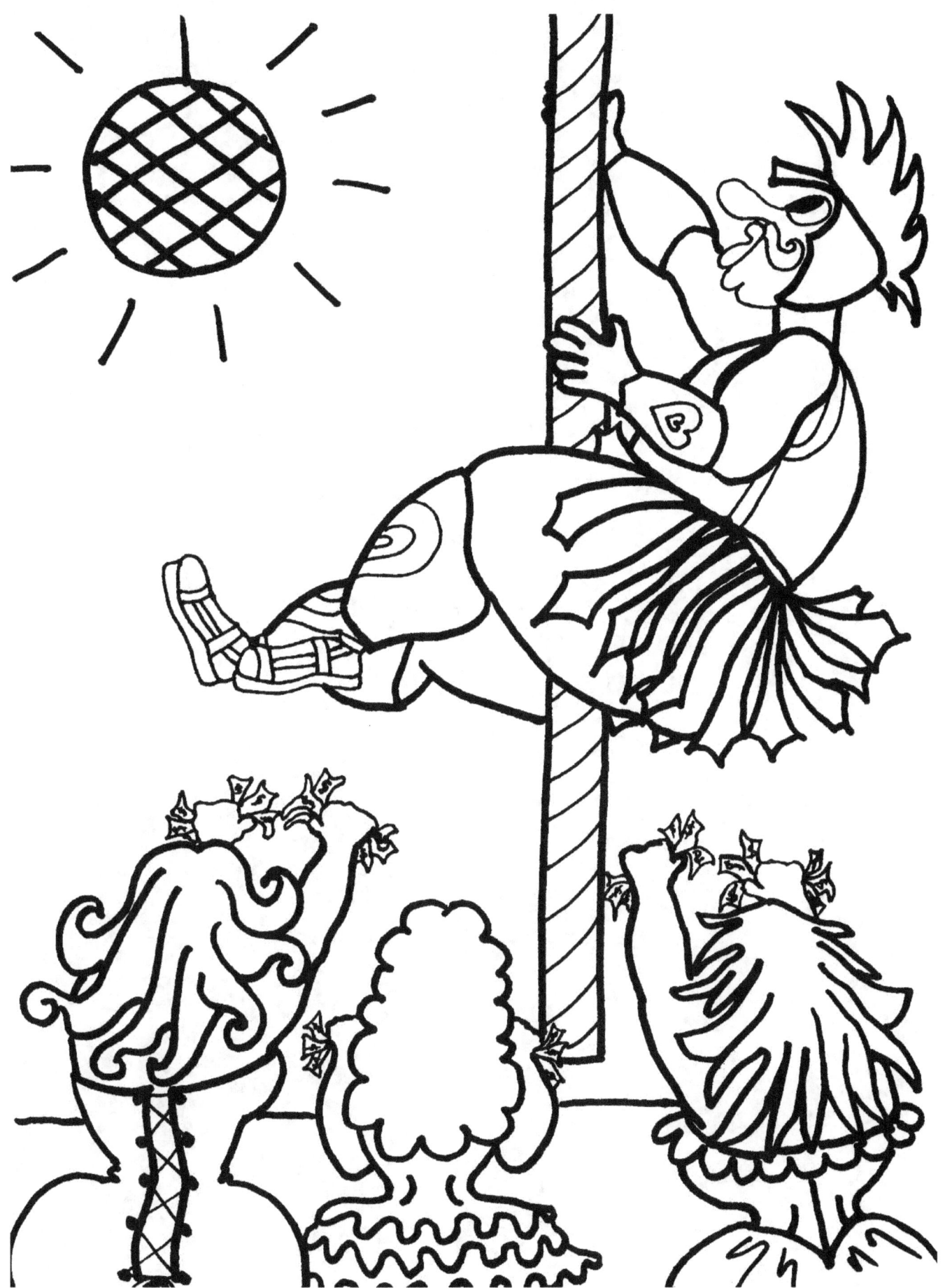

SPREAD EAGLE

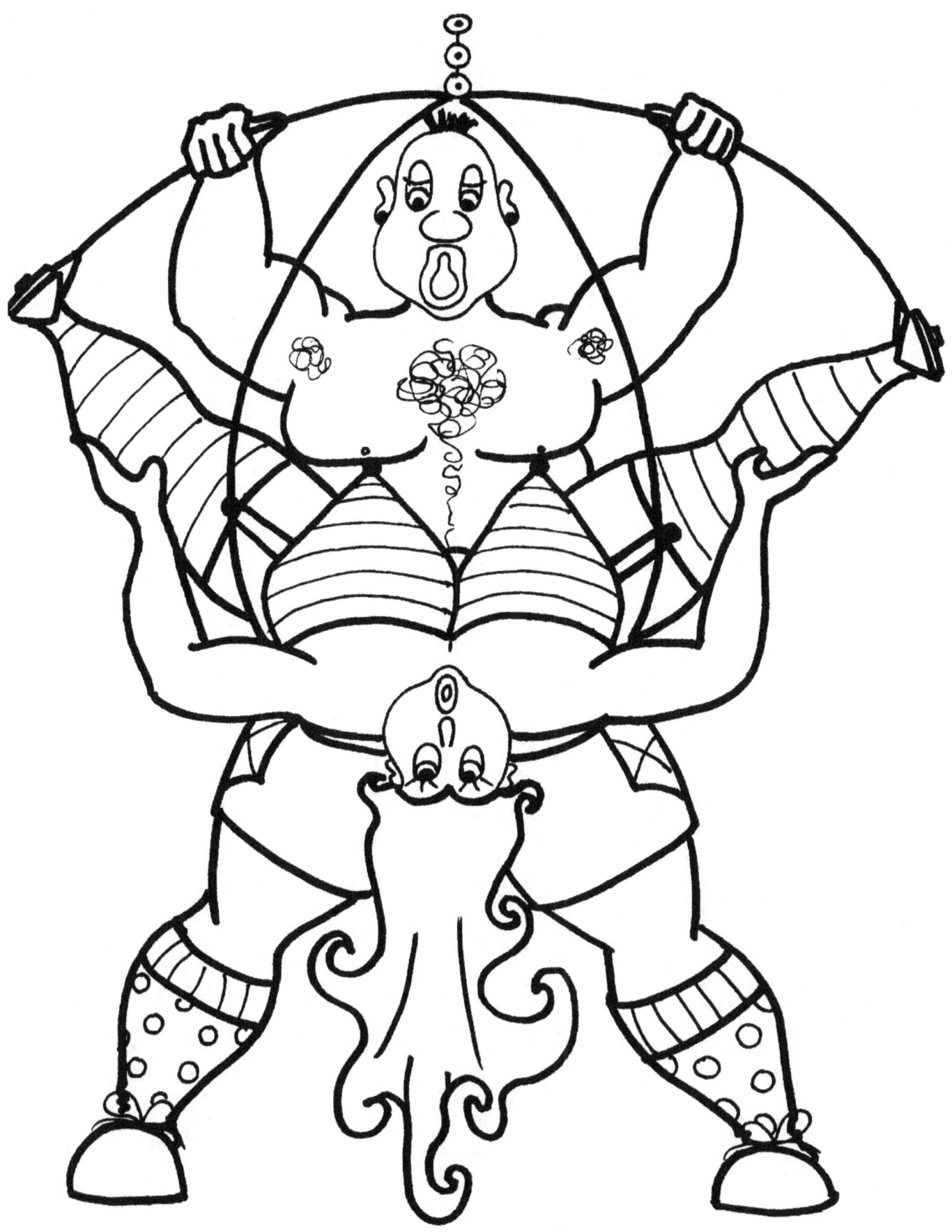

ABOUT THE AUTHOR

Alison Galvan is an award winning artist whose work is collected through galleries and online by art lovers from around the world. Originally from British Columbia, Canada, today Alison resides in Ontario where she and her husband are planning their next adventures now that their children are grown and have flown the coup.
For a full list of all Chubby Art Cartoon Colouring Books, check out
www.chubbyartcaratoons.com

www.ingramcontent.com/pod-product-compliance
Lightning Source LLC
Chambersburg PA
CBHW080831310526
45788CB00019B/3172